BAD BREATH
PERMANENT REMEDY

"Say Goodbye to Halitosis" Your Comprehensive modern proven Guide Book on Overcoming Bad Breath in both Kids and Adults

By

Dr. Suman Hashmi Das

TABLE OF CONTENT

CHAPTER 1

INTRODUCTION

Halitosis, or bad breath, can be a big deal, particularly right before you cuddle up with your significant other or whisper a joke to a friend. The good news is that by following a few easy steps, bad breath can often be avoided. Odor-producing bacteria that proliferate in the mouth are the source of bad breath. Bacteria grow on food particles left in your mouth and in the spaces between your teeth when you don't brush and floss on a regular basis. Your breath smells because these bacteria release sulfur compounds. Some foods, particularly those high in pungent oils like onions and garlic, can aggravate bad breath because the oils travel through your mouth and into your lungs. Another common cause of bad breath is smoking.

Halitosis, another name for bad breath, can be uncomfortable and in rare circumstances even frightening. It makes sense that mouthwash, gum, mints, and other breath freshening products are piled high on store shelves. However, a lot of these products are merely Band-Aid solutions. This is a result of their failure to deal with the root of the issue.

Bad breath can result from a variety of habits, diseases, and foods. Keeping your teeth and mouth clean can often help reduce bad breath. See your dentist or another medical expert if you are unable to treat your bad breath on your own to ensure that it is not the result of a more serious illness.

WHAT IS HALITOSIS?

Breath with an unpleasant odor is referred to as bad breath, or halitosis. Because they have grown accustomed to the bad breath, those who suffer from it frequently are unaware of how awful it smells. For others, however, when their partner speaks, laughs, or exhales, it's a full blast.

Breath odor is the primary sign of halitosis, an oral health issue. The first step in treating this avoidable condition is typically determining what is causing the bad breath.

SOME NOT TRUE MYTHS ABOUT HALITOSIS

MYTH 1: *Using mouthwash will help to permanently eliminate bad breath.*

Bad breath is only momentarily eliminated by mouthwash. If you do use mouthwash, look for one with an American Dental Association (ADA) seal that is both plaque-reducing and antiseptic (kills the germs that cause bad breath) it's a good idea to look for dental products that are approved by the American Dental Association (ADA) when choosing which ones to add to your shopping cart. Additionally, get recommendations from your dentist.

MYTH 2: *You shouldn't have bad breath if you brush your teeth.*

The majority of people, in actuality, barely brush their teeth for thirty to forty-five seconds, which is insufficient. At least twice a day, you should brush your teeth for two minutes on each side in order to thoroughly clean all of their surfaces. Brush your tongue as well, as bacteria like to reside there. It's equally important to floss because food particles and dangerous plaque that get lodged between your teeth and gums cannot be removed by brushing alone.

MYTH 3: *You can tell when you have bad breath by inhaling into your hand.*

False! Your throat is used differently when breathing than it is when speaking. Speaking tends to release the odors from the back of your mouth, which is the source of bad breath; breathing alone cannot eliminate this effect. Furthermore, it might be difficult for someone to detect foul breath because we have a tendency to grow accustomed to our own preferences.

Make sure you're taking good care of your teeth and mouth if you're worried about bad breath. Certain sugar-free mints and gums can also momentarily cover up smells. Your bad breath might be the result of a medical condition like sinusitis or gum disease, even if you brush and floss correctly and get regular cleanings at the dentist. Should you have concerns, give your dentist or physician a call. If there's another reason for your foul breath, they can determine it and assist you in treating it.

CHAPTER 2

CAUSES OF BAD BREATH

Your mouth is where most bad breath begins. There are numerous potential reasons, such as:

NOT CLEANING YOUR TEETH AND MOUTH: *Approximately 90% of cases of true halitosis have the odor coming from the mouth. This condition is referred to as oral halitosis, intra-oral halitosis, or oral malodor.*

The most frequent causes are bad oral hygiene that leads to odor-producing biofilm on the back of the tongue or other parts of the mouth. High concentrations of unpleasant odors are produced as a result of this biofilm. The primary source of the odors is the disintegration of proteins into their constituent amino acids, which is then followed by the additional breakdown of some amino acids to generate odorous gases. Oral malodor is correlated with volatile sulfur compounds, which typically go down after a successful course of treatment. Though they are less frequent than the back of the tongue, other areas of the mouth could also add to the overall odor. These areas are abscesses, dirty dentures, food-impaction areas between teeth, faulty dental work, interdental and subgingival niches, and descending order of prevalence. Additionally, oral lesions from viral infections such as HPV and herpes simplex can aggravate bad breath.

Because of certain foods (like garlic, onions, meat, fish, and cheese), smoking, and alcohol consumption, the severity of bad breath can vary throughout the day.

Because the mouth is inactive and exposed to less oxygen during the night, the odor is typically stronger when one awakens ("morning breath"). Whether it is temporary or persistent, bad breath usually goes away after eating, drinking, brushing, flossing, or using a specific mouthwash. An additional type of bad breath that affects about 25% of people in varying degrees is chronic bad breath.

Food particles stay in your mouth and cause bad breath if you don't brush and floss on a regular basis. Plaque is a colorless, sticky layer of bacteria that accumulates on your teeth. Plaque can cause irritation to your gums if it is not removed. It may eventually result in pockets of plaque forming between your teeth and gums. Gingivitis is the term for gum disease's early stages. Periodontitis is a late-stage gum disease associated with bone loss. Bacteria that cause odors can also be trapped on your tongue. Food particles and bacteria that cause odors can also accumulate in dentures and other fixed or removable oral appliances like braces that are ill-fitting or improperly cleaned.

TONGUE: The tongue is where mouth-related halitosis is most frequently found. Eighty to ninety percent of cases of mouth-related bad breath are caused by bacteria that produce fatty acids and malodorous compounds. On the posterior dorsum of the tongue, where normal activity largely disturbs them, large amounts of naturally occurring bacteria are frequently found. Because of its dryness and lack of cleansing, this area of the tongue is a perfect home for anaerobic bacteria, which thrive under a layer of dead and living bacteria that is constantly accumulating on top of food particles, dead epithelial cells, postnasal drip, and other debris. The putrescent smell of indole, skatole, and polyamines or the "rotten egg" smell of volatile sulfur compounds (VSCs) like hydrogen sulfide, methyl mercaptan, allyl methyl sulfide, and dimethyl sulfide can be produced by the anaerobic respiration of these bacteria when they are left on the tongue. Tongue coating is not the same as the presence of bacteria that cause halitosis on the back of the tongue. The majority of people with and without halitosis have some degree of white tongue coating, and bacteria are imperceptible to the unaided eye. Though a "white tongue" is considered a sign of halitosis, a visible coating of white spots on the tongue does not always correspond to the back of the tongue. A white tongue is typically regarded in oral medicine as an indicator of multiple medical disorders. When compared to normal subjects, patients with periodontal disease had a six-fold higher prevalence of tongue coating. Additionally, it was demonstrated that halitosis patients had noticeably higher bacterial loads in this area when compared to non-halitosis patients.

FOOD: A bad odor may result from the food particles breaking down in and around your teeth, which can attract more bacteria. Garlic, onions, and other foods high in spices can also contribute to bad breath. These foods affect your breath after they enter your bloodstream and travel to your lungs after being digested.

GUMMY/GUMS: Small groves between teeth and gums are known as gingival crevices, and they exist in healthy teeth, though gingivitis can cause them to swell. The depth of a periodontal pocket is greater than 3 mm; whereas the gingival crevice is less than 3 mm. usually gum disease (periodontitis) is accompanied by periodontal pockets. Regarding periodontal diseases' contribution to bad breath, there is some disagreement. But a common cause of severe halitosis is advanced periodontal disease. An increased risk of multiple gingival and periodontal abscesses is seen in people with uncontrolled diabetes. Large pockets where pus builds up are clearly visible in their gums. Bad breath could potentially originate from this nidus of infection. There is significant improvement in mouth odor when the subgingival calculus (hard plaque, or tartar) and friable tissue are removed. The process involves applying an antibiotic mouth rinse, scaling the gingiva, and planning the roots. Gram negative bacteria with the ability to produce VSC are the ones that cause periodontal disease and gingivitis, also known as periodontopathogens. When gingivitis and periodontal disease cause halitosis, methyl mercaptan is known to be the main contributing volatile sugar. It has been demonstrated that the amount of VSC on breath positively correlates with the number, depth, and bleeding of periodontal pockets when a dental probe is used to examine them. In fact, it has been demonstrated that VSCs themselves may be a factor in the tissue damage and inflammation that characterize periodontal disease. That being said, not every patient with halitosis also has periodontal disease, nor does every patient with periodontal disease have halitosis. While halitosis is more common in periodontal disease patients than in the general population, research has shown that the degree of tongue coating is more strongly correlated with halitosis symptoms than periodontal disease severity. A bad taste is another sign of periodontal disease, though it doesn't always go along with an odor that other people can smell.

MOUTH FEELING PARCHED/DRIED: Saliva aids in mouth cleaning by removing impurities that lead to unpleasant odors. Bad breath may be accompanied by xerostomia, also known as dry mouth (zeer-o-STOE-me-uh), a condition in which saliva production is reduced. Sleep causes dry mouth, which contributes to "morning breath." If you sleep with your mouth open, it gets worse. Diseases and issues with the glands that produce saliva can be the cause of persistent dry mouth.

TONSIL: Occasionally, food particles lodge in the tonsils, which are situated at the back of the throat, and solidify into calcium deposits known as tonsil stones or tonsilloliths. The percentage of cases of halitosis attributed to tonsil disorders is a matter of debate. After the mouth, some people assert that the tonsils are the primary source of halitosis. A report stated that tonsils accounted for about 3% of cases of halitosis. Chronic caseous tonsillitis (cheese-like material can be exuded from the tonsillar crypt orifi), tonsillolithiasis (tonsil stones), and less frequently peritonsillar abscess, actinomycosis, fungating malignancies, chondroid choristoma, and inflammatory myofibroblastic tumor are conditions of the tonsils that may be associated with halitosis.

INFECTIONS IN THE MOUTH: Bad breath can result from surgical wounds from oral surgery, including tooth extractions, gum disease, and mouth sores.

CIGARETTE GOODS: Bad breath is a result of smoking. In addition, gum disease, another cause of foul breath, is more common in smokers. Cigarettes, cigars, smokeless tobacco, and snuff are examples of tobacco products that stain teeth and increase the body's risk of several diseases. But they also contribute to foul breath. Also, there is an increased risk for tobacco users for the following:

- Periodontal disease
- Loss of taste perception
- Gum irritation
- Oral cancer

STOMACH: Most researchers believe that the stomach is a very rare cause of bad breath. The esophagus is a closed, collapsed tube, and persistent gas or foul-smelling material coming from the stomach signals a health issue that will show more serious symptoms than just bad breath. Examples of these problems include reflux that is severe enough to be bringing up stomach contents or a fistula that separates the stomach and esophagus.

OTHER AILMENTS OF THE MOUTH, NOSE AND THROAT: Tonsil stones, also known as tonsilloliths, are tiny stones that grow in the tonsils and are covered in bacteria that can lead to bad breath. Postnasal drip can be caused by infections or persistent swelling in the throat, sinuses, or nose. This is the feeling that runs down the back of your throat from nasal secretions. Moreover, this illness may result in foul breath.

MEDICATIONS: Certain medications may cause dry mouth, which can result in foul breath. Other medications are broken down by the body, releasing chemicals that can be inhaled.

ADDITIONAL REASONS: Certain illnesses, like certain cancers, can give one's breath a peculiar smell. The same holds true for illnesses involving the body's conversion of food into energy. Bad breath can result from persistent heartburn, a sign of gastro esophageal reflux disease, or GERD. A foreign object, like food particles stuck in the nose, can give young children bad breath.

CAUSES OF BAD BREATH IN KIDS

As soon as your child opens their mouth to cuddle, you can smell something foul on their breath. You are not alone among parents who have to deal with their child's foul breath, regardless of how long it has been present. Really, 37.6% of the child participants in a 2014 study with bad breath (halitosis) had it, according to the International Journal of Dental Hygiene.

My toddler's breath smells awful. Why is that? When my child has bad breath and a white tongue, should I worry? My adolescent has halitosis; is there anything I can do about it? You know what, we have the answers! The common causes of bad breath in children, treatment options, and the appropriate time to see a pediatric dentist are all covered in this post.

COATING OF THE TONGUE: Are they having bad breath and a white tongue? The formation of a tongue coating is another highly typical cause of foul breath in young children, adolescents, and adults. The back third of the tongue is frequently where food particles, bacteria that cause odors and decaying skin cells become lodged. The smell of these things breaking down is not pleasant, as you can imagine.

Consequently, why would a youngster have foul breath and white tongue? The tongue has tiny bumps called papillae that are filled with gunk that gives the appearance of being white. Both your child's foul breath and the white coating on their tongue can be eliminated by having them brush their teeth every time.

VERY POOR ORAL HYGIENE: Inadequate dental hygiene is the most frequent cause of foul breath in children. When food particles and plaque—the sticky bacterial film that builds up on teeth—are not eliminated through regular brushing and flossing, the bacteria in the mouth have something to eat. They emit sulfur compounds that are volatile and smelly while they eat.

LOOSE FILLINGS OR CROWNS IN PEDIATRICS: Food and bacteria can become trapped beneath a dental crown or filling that is loose or damaged in your child. It should come as no surprise that this will give children halitosis.

A PIECE OF STUCK IN THE NOSE: An object lodged in the nose must be mentioned when discussing the causes of bad breath in toddlers. Young children frequently stuff food and toys up their noses, which can cause irritation, runny noses, and bad breath if the foreign body becomes lodged there. Get medical help as soon as possible if you believe your child has stuck something up their nose, along with a fever and dark green mucus.

BIG TONSILS: Children who have big tonsils or tonsils with deep pits may have foul-smelling breath. This occurs as a result of the tonsils acting as a magnet for food particles, bacteria, and secretions from the nose. Additionally, tonsilloliths, or tonsil stones, can form in the pits and release an odor when they break down.

HOW TO HELP A CHILD WITH BAD BREATH

It may be tempting to give your child breath mints or a breath strip if they have bad breath, but these solutions aren't very effective and merely cover up the issue. Although the exact cause of your child's halitosis may vary, the following tips and remedies for bad breath are generally effective:

Teach children to take care of their teeth: Make sure they floss once a day and brush their teeth for at least two minutes twice a day. Make sure your child is brushing all of the surfaces of their teeth, the gum line, and their tongue completely to remove any coating. You will need to brush and floss your baby or younger toddler in order to get rid of bad breath. Preschoolers and older toddlers can start brushing on their own, but until they are around 7 or 8 years old, you should watch over their oral hygiene routine.

Examine the depth of your child's breathing: In addition to bad breath, habitual mouth breathing can cause several issues with oral health. You can get advice from your pediatric dentist, who is an expert in dental habits, including mouth breathing.

Make sure your child drinks lots of water to stay hydrated: Water helps fight dry mouth and helps drive food particles, bacteria, and plaque away.

Never undervalue the influence of breakfast: Children who eat and drink in the morning have less morning breath and more saliva produced.

Continue eating a balanced, healthful diet: Additionally, indulge in sugary sweets and starchy foods like chips sparingly. Reducing your intake of sugars and starches will help prevent cavities and bad breath because these foods are highly preferred by oral bacteria.

Attend your child's routine dental checkups and cleanings: Your child's teeth and gums will be examined by the dentist to ensure they are in excellent condition. They will also examine any restorations your child may have, such as a filling or crown. Should the dentist find any problems, addressing them early on will simplify and lessen the need for invasive treatment, as well as stop halitosis from occurring. Not only does a cleaning help with bad breath, but it also removes hardened plaque and helps shield teeth from cavities and gingivitis.

Consult your child's pediatrician if their foul breath is being caused by a medical condition or medication: Treatment for the illness often stops halitosis in its tracks. It wouldn't hurt to check if your child can try an alternate medication if the medication causing their bad breath and dry mouth is bothering them.

Give children xylitol-containing sugarless gum to chew on after meals and snacks, or anytime their mouths feel dry: Although this isn't the best way to treat toddler bad breath, older children who refuse to swallow the gum or leave it in odd places may find it useful. Chewing gum increases saliva production in the mouth, which helps to wash away bad bacteria from the teeth like a bath. It is believed that xylitol reduces the quantity of bacteria and plaque, which in turn lowers the risk of cavities.

WHEN TO CONTACT PEDIATRIC DENTIST FOR A CHILD'S BAD BREATH

See your pediatric dentist if your child has bad breath, red, swollen, bleeding gums, or pain in their teeth. It's possible that your child needs dental care for a condition like gingivitis or a cavity. Contact your pediatrician if you have bad breath along with other symptoms, such as a fever. These are symptoms of infection, and treating conditions like strep throat will necessitate the use of antibiotics.

However, children's bad breath is usually not a serious medical concern. See if your child's breath gets better by trying our advice and solutions. Tell your child's dentist at their subsequent appointment if it doesn't.

CHAPTER 3

TYPICAL KINDS OF BAD BREATH

Your body's metabolic processes or issues with your mouth, digestive system, or both can cause bad breath. Let's examine some of the most prevalent foul breath odors and their potential causes in more detail.

BREATH WITH A FRUITY OR SWEET SCENT: Diabetic ketoacidosis is a dangerous health condition that can result from uncontrolled diabetes. It can also cause other symptoms, like fruity or sweet-smelling breath. Fasting and low-carb diets can occasionally result in altered tastes or smells in your breath. It's been described as metallic by some. The smell is pleasant to others. When you follow a low-carb diet, your body burns fat for fuel, causing your breath and urine to contain chemicals called ketones. Your breath may smell different as a result of the accumulation of ketones.

THE SMELL OF NAIL POLISH REMOVER IN ONE'S BREATH: Your body uses carbohydrates as fast-burning fuel. You aren't eating a lot of carbohydrates when you follow a low-carb diet, such as the keto or paleo programs. Consequently, your body starts burning fat that has been stored rather than carbohydrates, which can result in the production of acetone. The same substance that's in many nail polish removers is acetone. Acetone release can also be brought on by diabetes.

BREATH WITH A PUTRID OR FOUL ODOR (SUCH AS THAT OF DEATH OR TRASH): The reason behind your breath smelling like rotting tissue could be an abscess or infection in your mouth, throat, or lungs.

For instance, bronchiectasis, a disorder that thickens and widens your bronchial tubes (air passages), can result in excessive mucus that has a foul stench and recurrent respiratory infections. Inadequate fit of dentures, crowns, and orthodontic appliances can also cause food to get stuck in spaces. It may smell like decay due to bacterial growth and leftover food.

Similarly, inadequate oral health can result in:

✓ **Lesions**

✓ **Fistulas**

✓ **Cavities**

✓ **Ulcers**

These incision-like gaps have the ability to hold food that is rotting or release foul odors. Untreated periodontal disease (also known as gum disease) may be another factor. Breath that smells rotten or decayed is another symptom of granulomatosis. This is an uncommon inflammatory illness that affects your nose, kidneys, and blood vessels. Early detection makes it treatable, but if treatment is not received, the condition may worsen.

SOUR-SMELLING BREATH: The muscle that separates your esophagus from your stomach doesn't close correctly when you have gastroesophageal reflux disease (GERD). Consequently, the contents of your stomach may reflux into your mouth, throat, or esophagus. Your breath may occasionally smell sour, like partially digested food, if you have GERD.

BREATH WITH AN AMMONIA OR URINE ODOR: Azotemia is the term for breath that smells like urine or ammonia. Usually, this illness is brought on by injury or disease that damages your kidneys. The ammonia smell comes from chemicals building up inside your body when your kidneys are unable to eliminate enough nitrogen.

SMELL OF EXCREMENT IN THE BREATH: Breath odors may indicate that there is an obstruction obstructing the waste passageways in your intestines.

A blockage may also cause you to have bad breath and the following symptoms:

- ✓ **Distension**
- ✓ **Vomiting**
- ✓ **Twitching**

✓ **Sick feeling**

✓ **Diarrhea**

Due to the potentially fatal nature of a colon blockage, it's critical that you seek medical assistance as soon as you notice these symptoms.

UNPLEASANT-SMELLING BREATH: The breath of those suffering from liver disease, such as cirrhosis, smells peculiarly musty. When the liver isn't working properly, the body produces volatile organic compounds (VOCs), which give off the characteristic odor known as fetor hepaticus. The musty smell is thought to be mostly caused by dimethylsulfide.

SMELLS LIKE MAPLE SYRUP IN THE BREATH: Maple syrup urine disease is a condition where a person's breath or urine smells like caramelized sugar or maple syrup. It is caused by an inability to metabolize three types of amino acids: valine, isoleucine, and leucine. If this disease is not identified and treated in a timely manner, it may result in major health issues and developmental issues.

BREATH WITH A FOOT SWEAT SCENT: The proper breakdown of proteins is essential for your body to function properly. The specific type of enzyme that isn't functioning properly can cause your breath to smell different when your body doesn't produce enough of the right kinds of enzymes to break down amino acids. Babies with the genetic disorder isovaleric acidemia have an accumulation of leucine in their blood, which gives them a smell that some people describe as being like sweaty feet.

THE SMELL OF BOILED CABBAGE IN ONE'S BREATH: A genetic condition known as hypermethioninemia is brought on by an inability of the body to metabolize the amino acid methionine. It gives off a boiled cabbage odor that permeates both your breath and urine. Other than this type of halitosis, people with this condition frequently don't have any other symptoms.

FISHY-SMELLING BREATH: Trimethylamine is an organic compound that your body is unable to break down; this condition is known as trimethylaminuria. This may give off an unpleasant odor to your breath, perspiration, and other body fluids.

RISK FACTORS LINKED TO BAD BREATH

Eat foods like garlic, onions, and spices, which are known to cause bad breath, and your risk of developing bad breath increases. There are a number of factors that can contribute to dry mouth, oral infections, diseases, smoking, and not cleaning your mouth well. Furthermore, bad breath may result from other illnesses like cancer or GERD.

WHAT IT MEANS TO ALWAYS HAVE BAD BREATH

Chronic halitosis may indicate the presence of gum disease. However, this isn't always the case. Additionally, halitosis may be a sign of any of the illnesses mentioned in the previous section.

Make an appointment with your dentist if you experience persistent bad breath. A periodontal (gum) procedure or dental cleaning should be helpful if halitosis is caused by inadequate oral hygiene. If your gums and teeth are in good condition, halitosis might be related to a problem in another area of your body.

CHAPTER 4

DIAGNOSIS OF BAD BREATH

The likelihood is that your dentist will rate the odor on a scale after smelling both your nose and mouth breath. Your dentist might scrape the back of your tongue to assess its odor, as this is where the smell usually originates. Certain chemicals responsible for bad breath can also be detected by certain devices. But sometimes these resources aren't accessible.

SELF DIAGNOSIS OF BAD BREATH

Although many people with bad breath can detect it in others, scientists have long believed that the smell of one's own breath is often difficult to detect due to acclimatization. According to research, our preconceived ideas about how bad halitosis should be make it difficult to evaluate oneself. Bad taste (metallic, sour, fecal, etc.) is a poor indicator of bad breath, despite the fact that some people believe it to be the cause. A close friend is frequently asked by patients to self-diagnose.

Licking the back of the wrist, letting the saliva dry for a minute or two, and then smelling the result is a common at-home technique for detecting bad breath. Research has shown that this test causes overestimation and should be avoided. A better method would be to use a plastic disposable spoon to gently scrape the back of the tongues posterior and then smell the drying residue. There are now home tests that use a chemical reaction to check tongue swabs for sulfur compounds and polyamines;

however, few studies have shown how well these tests actually detect the odor. Furthermore, multiple testing sessions are required because the intensity of breath odor varies throughout the day based on various factors.

TREATMENT OF BAD BREATH (HALITOSIS)

Treatment for halitosis is based on the underlying cause of the problem. For instance, better oral hygiene practices at home and a dental cleaning can probably help if bad breath is the result of poor oral hygiene. However, if halitosis is a sign of a different illness in another part of your body, your primary care physician can assist you with a correct diagnosis and course of action. Sometimes, in order to fight specific bacteria in your mouth, your dentist might suggest using particular mouth rinses.

Maintaining regular dental hygiene can help prevent cavities, minimize bad breath, and reduce the risk of gum disease. There are several ways to treat foul breath further. You'll probably need to see a specialist or your primary care physician if your dentist believes that there is another medical condition causing your bad breath. To help you better manage foul breath brought on by oral health problems, your dentist will collaborate with you. Dental interventions could involve:

- **TOOTHPASTES AND MOUTHWASHES:** Your dentist might suggest a mouthwash that eliminates bacteria if the accumulation of plaque on your teeth is the cause of your bad breath. In order to destroy the bacteria that cause plaque buildup, your dentist might also suggest toothpaste with an antibacterial ingredient.

- **THERAPY FOR DENTAL CONDITIONS:** Your dentist might advise you to see a periodontist, a specialist in gum disease treatment, if you have the condition. Gum disease can cause your gums to recede from your teeth, creating deep pockets that harbor bacteria that produce bad breath. These bacteria can occasionally only be eliminated by expert cleaning. Additionally, your dentist may advise replacing defective fillings, which serve as a haven for bacteria.

Treatment of halitosis can also depend on the following condition:

SIGNIFICANT PLAQUE ACCUMULATION: An antimicrobial mouthwash may be advised by your periodontist or dentist. In order to help get rid of bacteria that causes odor, you might also be instructed to gently brush your tongue after brushing your teeth.

HEALTH ISSUE: Treating and diagnosing an underlying medical issue may resolve bad breath.

IMPROPER ORAL HYGIENE: Your dentist will typically address the root of the issue if your foul breath is the result of poor oral hygiene.

GUM DISEASE: Your dentist may be able to treat gum disease if that is the underlying cause. Alternatively, a referral to an oral specialist—typically a periodontist may be made. The bacteria and tartar or plaque that have accumulated and are causing inflammation at the gum line are frequently removed with the aid of a periodontal cleaning.

PREVENTION OF BAD BREATH

To lessen or avoid foul breath:

Maintain clean mouth guards, retainers, dentures, and bridges: Clean your denture or bridge thoroughly at least once a day, or as instructed by your dentist, if you wear one. Make sure to clean any mouth guards or dental retainers you may have before using them. The best cleaning solution can be recommended by your dentist.

Maintain a moist mouth: Avoid tobacco use and sip lots of water. Limit your intake of alcohol, caffeine, and spicy foods. They can all cause mouth dryness. To produce more saliva, chew gum or bite into some candy, preferably sugar-free. Your doctor may recommend an artificial saliva substitute or an oral medication to increase salivary flow if you have persistent dry mouth.

After eating, give your teeth a brush: Have a toothbrush on hand at work for use after meals. Make sure to use toothpaste that contains fluoride at least twice a day, particularly after meals. It has been demonstrated that antibacterial toothpaste lessens foul breath.

At least once a day try and floss: By effectively cleaning the spaces between your teeth of food particles and plaque, proper flossing helps reduce bad breath.

Modify your food intake: Avoid foods that can cause bad breath, such as garlic and onions. Another factor associated with bad breath is eating a lot of sugary foods.

Change out your toothbrush: Replace your toothbrush every three to four months or sooner if necessary, when it starts to fray. Select a toothbrush with soft bristles as well.

Make time for routine dental exams: Generally speaking, you should visit the dentist twice a year. Your dentist can examine and clean your teeth or dentures during these examinations.

Grasp your tongue: Because your tongue harbors bacteria, gently brushing it can help lessen odors. For those with a tongue coated due to a significant bacterial overgrowth from smoking or dry mouth, for example—a tongue scraper could be helpful. Alternately, use a toothbrush with an integrated tongue cleaner.

Increase saliva production by chewing on sugar-free gum: sucking on sugar-free candies, or consuming nutritious foods that need a lot of chewing. Products that can help your body produce saliva or create artificial saliva may be suggested or prescribed by your dentist.

CHAPTER 5

BEST TECHNIQUES FOR BRUSHING THE TEETH

Here are some pointers and methods for doing a thorough tooth brushing:

- ✓ Apply a toothbrush with soft bristles. Make sure you can reach every part of your mouth with its size and shape.

- ✓ At the very least, change your toothbrush every three to four months or more frequently if it appears worn.

- ✓ Use short strokes with your toothbrush, about the width of a tooth, and hold it at a 45-degree angle toward your gums. Make sure you brush every tooth, including the top, inside, and outside.

✓ Don't apply too much pressure to your brush. Gum recession may result from vigorous brushing or from using a brush with firm bristles.

BEST TECHNIQUES FOR FLOSSING THE TEETH

Brushing is not the only thing that counts interdental cleaning is too. Where your toothbrush cannot reach, floss can reach. To correctly floss:

✓ Cut a length of floss, about eighteen inches long, and wrap it around your middle fingers.

✓ Hold the floss firmly between your fingers, an inch or two between them, using your thumbs and forefingers.

✓ The floss should be guided between the middle sections of your teeth. It should then be wrapped around one tooth in a "C" shape and rubbed seven to ten times along its length. (Note: Plaque cannot be removed from the surfaces of your teeth without friction. Large food particles and debris can be effectively removed with water flossers. However, make sure to use regular floss in addition to your water flosser.)

✓ Repeat these actions while wrapping the floss around the adjacent tooth.

For the first few days, if you haven't been flossing, you may experience some bleeding and discomfort, but those should go away.

WHEN SHOULD I SEE MY DENTIST?

Make an appointment with your dentist if you maintain good hygiene but still have halitosis. Plaque may simply accumulate more quickly in some people and require more frequent cleanings. To find out if gum disease is the reason for your halitosis, you can also make an appointment with a periodontist, a specialist in gum disease. Your primary care physician can identify whether halitosis is being caused by another condition if your dentist is unable to find any oral health issues, such as cavities or gum disease.

PREPARING FOR YOUR DENTIST'S APPOINTMENT

These suggestions may be helpful if you're visiting your dentist regarding foul breath:

✓ When testing for bad breath, dentists typically prefer morning appointments. This lessens the possibility that anything you eat during the day will have an impact on the test.

✓ For your appointment, avoid wearing scented lotions, lipsticks, or lip gloss. These goods could cover up any smells.

✓ Consult your dentist to determine whether you need to reschedule your appointment if you have taken antibiotics in the past month.

WHAT TO ANTICIPATE FROM YOUR DENTIST

Most likely, your dentist will begin by enquiring about your health history using inquiries like these:

- ✓ Do you suffer from sinus issues or allergies?
- ✓ What do you believe could be the source of your foul breath?
- ✓ Has your foul breath been noted and commented upon by others?
- ✓ When did your foul breath start to occur?
- ✓ Is your breath foul-smelling occasionally or consistently?
- ✓ How frequently do you clean your dentures or brush your teeth?
- ✓ How frequently do you floss?

- ✓ Which food types do you typically eat?

- ✓ What vitamins and medications do you take?

- ✓ What medical conditions do you suffer from?

- ✓ Do you primarily use your mouth to breathe?

- ✓ Are you a snorer?

To maximize the duration of your appointment, prepare responses to these questions.

CHAPTER 6

HOW TO SMELL YOUR OWN BREATH

Almost everyone worries about the smell of their breath at least occasionally. Your perception that your breath is unpleasant may be accurate if you recently consumed something spicy or woke up with cotton mouth. That being said, it can be difficult to accurately detect bad breath, or halitosis, by simply sniffing at your own breath.

It's difficult to detect your own breath odor, so people with bad breath sometimes believe they don't have it while those without it frequently mistakenly believe they do. Sometimes referred to as the "bad breath paradox," this is the inability to accurately determine whether or not your breath smells. Here, we'll talk about possible causes of bad breath, how to prevent it, and whether you can measure your own bad breath.

CAN YOU SMELL YOUR OWN BREATH?

The reason why it's difficult to smell your own breath is not entirely understood. However, the ability of your sensory nervous system to adapt to the constantly shifting stimuli around you may be the basis for this phenomenon. We call this sensory adaptation.

Your five senses are how sensory information enters your body. These are:

- ✓ **Aroma**
- ✓ **Listening**
- ✓ **Flavor**
- ✓ **Contact**

✓ Vision

Your nose is an excellent tool for distinguishing between noxious smells, like smoke, and olfactory cues, like the aroma of cooking your favorite dish. As your sense of smell adjusts to new stimuli, familiar scents tend to lose their intensity and fade into the background, as long as they are not harmful. Because you always smell your own breath and it doesn't hurt you, you grow used to the smell and eventually stop smelling it. Anatomy may also play a role in the incapacity to detect your own breath. An orifice located at the back of the mouth facilitates communication between the nose and mouth. It might be difficult for you to detect your own breath precisely as a result.

HOW TO GIVE IT A GO

The classic "breathe in your hand and smell it" method is probably not new to you if you've ever watched a movie about awkward teenagers. Hollywood's interpretation of the matter notwithstanding, this method is not very precise. Using your tongue to lick the inside of your wrist and inhale is a more accurate manual breath test. Your nose will have an easier time detecting the smell of breath on skin. Nevertheless, there is some uncertainty with this method.

ALTERNATIVE METHODS TO FIND OUT

To find out whether your breath smells, you can try a few more techniques like the following:

AT HOME: Get a reliable person to tell you whether your breath smells good or bad. Assessing and getting rid of bad breath can both benefit from using a tongue scraper. Smell the scraper and scrape the back of your tongue, which is frequently the cause of foul breath. Include using a scraper or a toothbrush to brush your tongue every day if it smells bad in your oral hygiene regimen.

IN THE DENTAL OFFICE: You can also request a bad breath test from your dentist. There are various kinds:

- ✓ *HALIMETER MEASUREMENT:* The volatile sulfur compound (VSC) level is determined by this test. Bacteria overgrowth in the mouth or intestines is the cause of VSCs. Parts per billion of VSCs are measured using halimeter tests. Smelly breath is usually indicated by measurements above 100 parts per billion. Customers can also purchase and utilize halimeter tests. There are a few that are more trustworthy than others. Find out which one your dentist recommends before making a purchase.

✓ **ORGANOLEPTIC TECHNIQUE:** This method uses a plastic straw to allow a dentist to personally evaluate how your breath smells. For the purpose of diagnosis, the dentist will frequently compare nasal and oral exhalations. These tests might occasionally be in conflict with one another. Consult your dentist about the most appropriate test type for you.

A BRIEF SUMMARY

A common condition that can lead to low self-esteem or embarrassment is halitosis. Yet having foul breath is not a reason for embarrassment. Frequently, it's just your body's way of alerting you to an irregularity. The good news is that treating the underlying medical condition is usually enough to eliminate halitosis. Together, your primary care physician and dentist can determine what is best for you.

NOTE:

- ✓ Bacteria that produce sulfur in the tongue and throat are the cause of halitosis.
- ✓ The main culprits are foods that cause dry mouth, smoking, not brushing your teeth properly, and having a coated tongue.

✓ The underlying cause of halitosis will determine how it is treated.

FAQs ABOUT BAD BREATH (HALITOSIS)

WHAT PRECISELY IS FOUL BREATH? An oral stench that is stronger than what is considered socially acceptable is called halitosis. This ailment is a symptom with multiple underlying causes rather than a disease. Two types of bad breath exist: chronic bad breath and occasional or transient bad breath. Most people briefly go through halitosis; this is caused by eating foods high in aroma and smoking tobacco. Conversely, an underlying illness or microbial deterioration in your mouth is the causes of chronic halitosis.

IN WHAT WAYS CAN FOUL BREATH BE AVOIDED OR TREATED? If you maintain good dental hygiene and halitosis still occurs, the tongue is probably the source of the odor. You might require tongue cleaning. Cleaning dentures or bridges at least once a day is advised if you have them. To lessen halitosis, it would also be beneficial to drink lots of water and cut back on alcohol and coffee.

WHICH FACTORS FREQUENTLY CONTRIBUTE TO FOUL BREATH? The coating of the tongue is the most frequent cause of halitosis. This is because your tongue's upper surface provides an optimal environment for the growth of bacteria. Food debris buildup, poor oral hygiene, dental plaque, and cavities can also cause bad breath. It has also been demonstrated that unclean dentures can aggravate bad breath. In addition to these, common causes include gum disease, periodontitis, tonsillitis, and xerostomia (dry mouth).

My breath seems awful a lot of the time, not only in the morning. TO WHAT EXTENT IS THIS UNCOMMON ISSUE? Halitosis, also known as persistent bad breath, is a very common complaint that is estimated to affect millions of people, with 25 to 50 percent of middle-aged and older adults being affected. At an estimated $3 billion a year, it is the primary driver of the breath mint and mouth rinse markets. It's also the third most common reason (after gum disease and tooth decay) for which people visit the dentist. Thus, you are not alone if you suffer from bad breath.

DO SOURCES OTHER THAN THE MOUTH CAUSE BAD BREATH? Foul-smelling substance called volatile sulfur compounds (VSCs) is often the source of bad breath, which is most often the result of oral activity. On the other hand, it could originate from the nose, potentially due to a foreign body or sinus infection. Halitosis may occasionally be brought on by tonsil pus. Some illnesses can also cause your breath to occasionally smell bad.

WHAT HABIT CAN CAUSE BAD BREATH? Tobacco usage is one of the worst habits when it comes to bad breath. Your mouth will taste and smell like an ashtray from the simple act of smoking alone, not to mention the health risks involved. An excessively sweet diet is also counterproductive because it feeds the natural bacteria in your mouth, which then builds up to decorate your teeth and gums with bacteria. With your body producing more ammonia in an attempt to try and metabolize food, diets that cut carbohydrates can often double your chances of developing bad breath. A different kind of risk exists for those who fast or skip meals frequently because chewing produces saliva, which keeps your mouth from drying out and smelling bad. Breath odors can develop when you stop for extended periods of time. Those who frequently breathe through their mouths are also affected by dry mouth, which puts them in the unfortunate position of having foul breath. Ultimately, having bad breath can result from excessive stress.

ARE UNDERLYING HEALTH PROBLEMS SIGNIFICANT BY BAD BREATH? Indeed, a recurrent case of bad breath could result from other medical conditions. Acid reflux and heartburn are common conditions that can cause bad taste in the mouth. In other situations, the problem might be caused by bacteria and mucus accumulation from a sinus infection. Diabetes can be detected by slightly fruity breath that isn't overtly pleasant or offensive, and kidney disease can be indicated by a strong ammonia smell.

Bad breath can result from periodontal diseases like gingivitis, which are caused by an overabundance of bacteria in the mouth. Furthermore, your mouth is unable to naturally remove food particles and bacteria from your teeth and gums before they decompose and begin to decay due to dry mouth, which lowers saliva production. See your dentist if your bad breath seems to indicate a more serious problem or if you can't seem to control it with brushing, flossing, and rinsing.

DOES CHEWING GUM ASSIST IN QUITTING HARMFUL BREATH? Both yes and no: Since dry mouth is frequently the cause of bad breath, chewing sugar-free gum can be a great way to stimulate saliva production. Saliva not only helps wash away bacteria but also draws unwanted food particles out of your mouth before they have a chance to decompose. Nonetheless, sugar-filled gums, candies, and mints won't be helpful. They might cover up the smell, but they won't really get rid of the bacteria making your breath smell. This is due to the fact that sugar adheres to your teeth and gums, where it can decompose and produce more odor and plaque. Increased plaque causes even worse breath. The best course of action is to rinse, brush, and floss twice a day. It will guarantee that your mouth is as clean as possible.

HOW CAN I DETERMINE IF MY BREATH IS FOUL? There are numerous subtle indicators that indicate bad breath. Have you ever noticed that when you start talking, people move away? There's a quick test you can take if you suspect you have bad breath. You can pretty much guarantee that your breath is bad if you lick the inside of your unscented wrist and take a sniff. Alternatively, get an honest answer from a very close friend, but make sure they are a true friend first.

WHAT ASSISTANCE CAN MY DENTIST PROVIDE? The most common cause of bad breath is gum disease. The bacteria that cause it are found in tartar, which is calcified plaque, and plaque, which are the soft deposits that accumulate on your teeth. During a routine examination, your dentist will be able to evaluate the condition of your gums and determine whether this is the reason. It might then be suggested that you schedule several appointments to see the hygienist. In addition to helping you learn the best oral hygiene practices, she or he will treat the issue by removing both soft and hard deposits from your teeth. Make an appointment with us to discuss how we can assist.

HOW CAN I INFORM SOMEONE THAT THEY SMELL BAD? We've all probably encountered someone with foul breath, but very few people are willing to talk about it. Telling someone they have bad breath is obviously a very delicate matter. You never know, they might never talk to you again if they feel offended or embarrassed! It's important to keep in mind, though, that a variety of issues could be the cause of bad breath. Acknowledging their foul breath allows the person to address the underlying cause. If the person has a medical condition that is currently being treated, it might be the cause of their bad breath. You could try speaking with their partner or family member. You could print a copy of this page and place it in a visible location for the person in question. It's important to keep in mind that oral malodor is a severe social problem that occasionally signals a medical problem. That is treatable, though, which is good news!

WHICH PRODUCTS ARE OFFERED? Specialty oral care products are widely available and include toothpaste, mouth rinse, and spray forms. You'll have cleaner teeth, better breath, and the self-assurance to smile all day long if you use these. The purpose of these products is to get rid of odor-causing substances, not cover them up. For more information, ask your dentist. As part of a regular oral hygiene routine, the specialty products' safe, potent antibacterial formula fights plaque and helps maintain a fresh, clean, and healthy mouth.

✓ ***Rinses of the mouth:*** We advise using mouthwash without alcohol, whether it is flavored or not. Rinse twice a day with 10ml for one minute; do not rinse with water afterward. The majority of mouthwashes are made to last up to eight hours.

- ✓ *Sprays for the mouth:* Are handy to have in your pocket, purse, car, or anywhere you want the comfort of clean breath when you aren't near the restroom.

- ✓ *Toothpaste:* Gritty toothpaste brands aid in removing more tartar and plaque. To guarantee decay prevention, buy those with a minimum fluoride content of 1450 ppm.

- ✓ *Sugar-Free Chewing Gum:* Gum helps to increase saliva production, which lessens bad breath. It also leaves behind a fresh, minty scent.

www.ingramcontent.com/pod-product-compliance
Lightning Source LLC
Chambersburg PA
CBHW071102290526
45795CB00004B/1624